A Step-By-Step Guide

How to Tell Food
WHO'S BOSS

Lorie Eber

Dedication

I want to thank my trusted support team for helping me get this book to print. The stalwarts are Judy Rose, who catches all my grammatical errors and typos, and Victoria Vinton, who makes my words look pretty on the page.

I also want to acknowledge my life partner and biggest cheerleader, my devoted husband, Wes. I never expected to be blessed with a companion with whom I have a mind meld, but life is full of surprises. He enriches my life more every day.

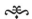

Contents

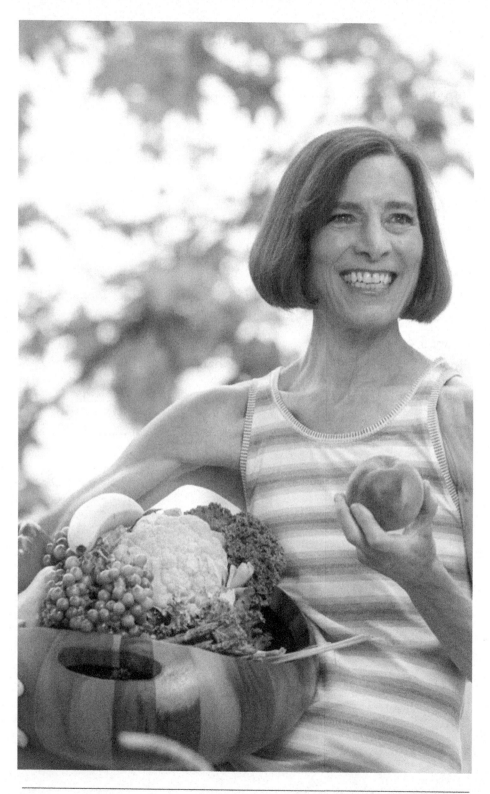

How to Show Food Who's Boss

Introduction

Do you feel that you have most parts of your life under control but that your eating habits remain mysteriously untamed? Do you experience days when you think about the food you downed rushing from one appointment to another and know that you deserve a butt kicking? Would you like to tell food who's boss and finally get this important part of life under control?

There are many reasons why maintaining a healthy weight and not joining the ranks of the 74% of adults in the U.S. who are overweight or obese is a discouragingly difficult undertaking. The fact that 90% of dieters regain the lost weight demonstrates the arduousness of the task. The sad irony is that it just shouldn't be so hard since no one shoves the food in our mouths. We are responsible for all the food choices we make, whether they be healthy, unhealthy, or somewhere in-between.

While I have all kinds of Nutrition and Wellness Coaching certifications, mostly what I do is get inside my clients' heads and try to figure out how their thinking and emotions affect their food choices and overall eating patterns. Essentially a good Nutritionist is an "amateur shrink." That skill reigns supreme because changing your diet is more about changing your mindset than anything else. No super-food, fat burner pill, or celebrity regimen will get you there. And since we have yet to develop the technology for an instantaneous brain make-over, behavior change necessarily takes time. "Short cuts" turn out to be the long way around.

In this book, I'll explore the multitude of reasons why the vast majority of Americans are carrying around more girth than the structure God gave them can bear. I'll also delve into the brain work that needs to be done to control the mouth. Extricating yourself from eating on auto-pilot or in response to unrecognized social pressure, and beginning to acknowledge what your food intake looks like on a daily basis, are the first steps on the bumpy road to acquiring new health habits. Unfortunately, when you decide to embark on the journey to a healthy life, all the tempting drive-thrus and restaurants remain open, continuing to beckon you to come by. This is where the development of new skills is necessary. This book will provide you with the tools you need to tell food who's boss and live a healthy lifestyle that makes you feel energetic and in control.

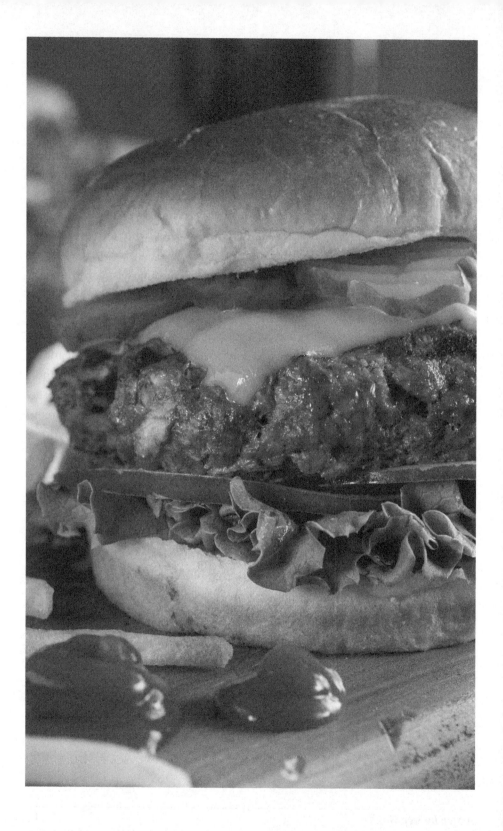

1

How Your Brain Undermines Your Good Intentions

Does This Sound Familiar?

You have a crazy life and eating is spur of the moment, mostly drive-thru and DoorDash. Your preferences go towards cheeseburgers and fries or tacos. You also have a sweet tooth and shop Trader Joe's® regularly to stock up on JoeJoe's. You look forward to fall when Starbucks® releases its Pumpkin Spice Frappuccino.

While this diet is super-enjoyable, you know that it's the reason the number on the scale is slowly creeping up. That's starting to nag at you. You really don't have a ready answer, so you Google "best diets" and come up with Keto and Intermittent Fasting. You end up trying both of them and lose a little weight, but sadly it all comes back on. Next you decide to just "be good" and that lasts until Wednesday when your girlfriend wants to splurge at the Cheesecake Factory®. You overindulge and feel terrible afterwards.

While commiserating with some friends, one suggests you all go on a 7-Day Detox Diet together. You're desperate enough to go for it and starve yourself on juices and teas until you reach for that carton of Ben & Jerry's Cookie Dough® that you hid in the deep recesses of your freezer. You scarf it down in one sitting.

1. Your Brain is on Autopilot

You mean to change your eating habits, but you keep going back to the tried and true.

YOUR ACTIONS

- You momentarily entertain the idea of not getting the fries when you're ordering at the drive-thru, but at the last minute you tack them onto your order.
- You sit down with a bag of chips and tell yourself that for once, you won't finish the bag. But when you reach in for another chip, they're all gone.
- You think about ordering the turkey sub at Jersey Mike's® when you go out to get lunch, but then you remember how good the Reuben tastes.
- You vow not to grab a humongous cookie while you're waiting in line to pay for your healthy salad, but the wait is too long, you're starving, and can't resist.
- You know today is donut day at work and you decide to bring your breakfast so you can resist the treats. Then a co-worker walks by with a chocolate donut with sprinkles. It looks so yummy that you weaken.

YOUR RATIONALIZATIONS

- I know that if I get "the usual," I'll be satisfied.
- When I looked, almost all the chips were gone already, so why not finish them?
- I'll do better next time.
- The cookies were homemade and they smelled too good to resist.
- I ate a healthy breakfast so I deserve a little indulgence.
- Other reasons: _____

2. The Junk Food Smorgasbord Is Just Too Tempting

You try to avoid overeating but there's food everywhere.

YOUR ACTIONS

- You go to a Super Bowl party and try to "be good" but the vast array of chips and dips, wings, nachos, and cheeseburger sliders is impossible to resist.
- You're at a boring out-of-town conference and during the afternoon break you sample a chocolate chip cookie, grab a soda for a caffeine rush, and gobble down a few chocolates and just-made potato chips.
- You go to Costco starving and sample mini cheesecake, meatballs, and exotic cheeses.
- You go to a baby shower and are greeted by a panoply of blue and pink cupcakes, cake pops, blondies, and chocolate dipped pretzels. You dig in.
- You board a flight without bringing your own food and end up ordering a snack box consisting of white cheddar puffs, honey mustard pretzels, gummi bears, and OREO® cookies.

YOUR RATIONALIZATIONS

- The Super Bowl spread looks so yummy and if there's any day to be a bit indulgent, it's today.
- I'm falling asleep and I need caffeine and sugar to power thorough the rest of the afternoon.
- I can't rejesct my neighbor's kindness, and the treats smell delicious.
- Let's face it, the highlight of a baby shower is the fun, colorful desserts.
- I'm starving and this is what they offer on the flight.
- Other reasons: _____

3. Whatever is Quick and Easy Jumps into Your Mouth

Even when you plan to eat healthy, you often end up eating restaurant-prepared food.

YOUR ACTIONS

- You planned to make that healthy chicken marsala recipe you found over the weekend, but when you get home, the leftover Chinese takeout jumps onto your plate.
- You meant to get up in time to eat an omelet with veggies, but you had to clean up the dog's mess, so you went to Dunkin' Donuts™ and got a large latte and a blueberry muffin.
- You forgot to bring your lunch to work and intended to go to the poke place to get a healthy meal, but your co-workers decided to go to In N Out™ and you couldn't say no.
- You intended to have chicken and veggies for dinner but you realized that you forgot to defrost the chicken so you DoorDash pizza instead.
- You meant to eat the leftover stew you made but you ended up getting home late and dealing with your sister's issues and were so mentally exhausted you decided you needed to eat the leftover cake for dinner.

YOUR RATIONALIZATIONS

- I'm way too tired to cook and the takeout will just go to waste if I don't eat it.
- After the rude awakening, I deserve a warm muffin.
- I'll be good and bring my lunch tomorrow.
- DoorDashing pizza is so easy, plus it's cheap and yummy.
- I'm upset and leftovers don't fit the bill, but chocolate cake does.
- Other reasons: _____

4. Eating is the Highlight of Your Days

You know you should eat healthy, but every event and social gathering is a food fest.

YOUR ACTIONS

- You retired recently and now plan your days around seeking out new restaurants, reading up on the chefs and trendy dishes, and eating out almost every night.
- You watch all the cooking shows, think about food constantly, and try your hand at whipping up the scrumptious meals you see the professionals prepare.
- You absolutely hate your job and organize a lunch group as soon as you get to the office in the morning.
- You and your husband seem to have evolved into a couple with totally separate lives and the only thing you really enjoy together anymore is eating out.
- You're a very social person with a lot of girlfriends who play bunco, shop and lunch together, and munch their way through book club.

YOUR RATIONALIZATIONS

- Restaurant research is a productive way to fill my day and I love discovering new places to go.
- Cooking is fun and creative and maybe I'll turn into the dinner party queen.
- If I choose where the group is going for lunch, we can avoid all the back and forth about restaurant selection.
- We might as well do something together and we both like eating.
- I want to stay social and that just involves a lot of eating.
- Other reasons: _____

5. You Exercise Your Emotions with Food

You try to stay on a healthy track, but when you're stressed or bored you can't resist comfort snacking.

YOUR ACTIONS

- You work all day and then leap into the mom role as soon as you get home, so you eat some chocolate as your "me time."
- You get bored during the day and head to the kitchen for chips or a bag of Flamin' Hot CHEETOS®.
- You're frustrated because you tried really hard but still got a "D" on your Calculus final, so you soothe yourself with Trader Joe's™ Dark Chocolate Peanut Butter Cups.
- You catch Covid and have to quarantine at home so you decide to Instacart the ingredients to whip up a batch of brown butter chocolate chunk cookies.
- You have a big presentation at work to tomorrow and feel super nervous, so you eat snacks instead of a healthy dinner.

YOUR RATIONALIZATIONS

- I deserve to do whatever I want after getting through a long day and I choose chocolate.
- Snacking relieves my boredom.
- Chocolate and peanut butter always make me feel better about myself.
- I feel lousy and making cookies always improves my mood.
- I can't focus enough to make a meal, but snacks are easy.
- Other reasons: _____

6. You Pride Yourself on Being a Foodie

Your reward for getting through a tough week is enjoying a scrumptious meal at one of your favorite restaurants.

YOUR ACTIONS

- You hate to cook so you eat out several times a week.
- You're a foodie and feel compelled to try out all the new restaurants.
- You go to the same restaurant once a week with your friends.
- You go on vacation with the goal of enjoying the local cuisine.
- You choose the restaurant when you go out with friends because you're the expert.

YOUR RATIONALIZATIONS

- I want to enjoy eating and my cooking doesn't make that happen.
- I love the adventure of trying a new restaurant.
- I get a kick out of walking into a restaurant where they know me and treat me special.
- I'm only going to visit this country once and eating like a native is part of the experience.
- I hate it when my friends can't decide where to eat so I just take charge.
- Other reasons: _____

7. You Neglect to Plan Your Food When You Think About Your Day

You get overwhelmed just planning what you need to do for your family and job every week and there never seems to be time to figure out a healthy eating plan.

YOUR ACTIONS

- You're so busy making breakfast and lunch for your kids that you don't eat until noon.
- You meant to plan the week's food on Sunday, but you never got to it.
- You have so much to do in the morning, packing a breakfast or lunch just isn't feasible.
- You intend to cook something for dinner but end up getting home late, so you stop at the drive-thru instead.
- You planned to make a chicken dish for dinner but forgot to defrost the meat.

YOUR RATIONALIZATIONS

- I have to get the kids fed and I'll worry about myself later.
- I know I should meal plan on Sunday, but doing errands takes up the whole day.
- I thought about taking food to the office today, but I couldn't because I just ran out of time.
- I ended up staying at the office late so there's no time to cook and I'm way too tired anyway.
- I meant to "be good" but with so much to do, taking the chicken out fell through the cracks.
- Other reasons: _____

8. You Let Yourself Get Starving

Somehow it seems that things always take longer than you antic-
ipated so you end up having to resort to the drive-thru because
you're starving.

YOUR ACTIONS

- You assume you'll be home in time for lunch, but it's 2:00 pm and you find the closest fast-food chain.
- You weren't hungry when you woke up, but by 11:30 am you're ravenous, so you go grab a burger and fries.
- You meant to bring your lunch but realize you left it at home on the counter.
- You do a lot of sampling while you're cooking dinner because you're starving.
- You're trying to eat healthy so you choose a salad for lunch, but head to the kitchen in search of a snack by mid-afternoon.

YOUR RATIONALIZATIONS

- I'd planned to throw together a sandwich at home, but I just wasn't able to get back there in time.
- I'm never hungry when I get up, so I try to wait until I'm hungry to eat.
- I was in a hurry so I just ran out of the house.
- I may sample a bit when I'm cooking, but I don't think it really amounts to much.
- I figure if I eat a salad for lunch, I'll lose weight.
- Other reasons: _____

9. All Your Friends are Foodies

Unfortunately all your friends are really into food and that makes it really hard not to overindulge.

YOUR ACTIONS

- You try a new trendy restaurant with your friends every week.
- You belong to a gourmet cooking club – indulgence is the whole point.
- You and your friends are always talking about the latest social media food buzz.
- You go on a girlfriend vacation that focuses on fine dining.
- You and your friends exchange pics of your latest scrumptious plates.

YOUR RATIONALIZATIONS

- I socialize by eating in trendy gourmet restaurants.
- I love discovering new flavor combinations with other like-minded friends.
- I relax by following my favorite foodies on YouTube and Instagram.
- If you can't splurge when you're on vacation, when can you?
- I love taking pics of gourmet meals and sharing them with my friends.
- Other reasons: _____

10. You Can't Quiet the Voices in Your Head

It seems like you spend far too many waking hours in food fantasy land.

YOUR ACTIONS

- You eat constantly because you can't stop thinking about food all the time.
- You spend the drive home from work thinking about what treat you'll reward yourself with, and you scarf down the cookies as soon as you get home.
- You need something to munch while you binge watch Netflix, so you grab the chips.
- You eat a huge dinner because the scale was down a little this morning.
- You're upset with yourself for overeating at the restaurant, so you just blow off the whole week.

YOUR RATIONALIZATIONS

- I can't help it; I just have a love affair with food.
- I earned those cookies because I had a horrendous day at work.
- I can't watch my shows without munching on something.
- I earned a little indulging by being so good all week.
- I already blew it, so I might as well enjoy the rest of the week and start over on Monday.
- Other reasons: _____

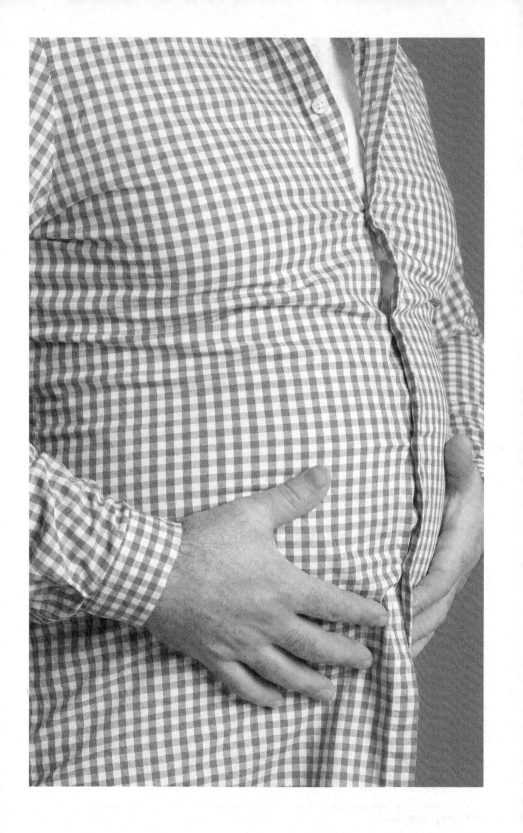

2

What Might Motivate You to Change Your Eating Habits?

Does This Sound Familiar?

You're inching up to retirement age and your two kids are now in college. Thank God! Those are the good things. The miserable thing is the 40 pounds that has crept on ever so steadily over the course of the last decade. Dozens of quick weight loss diets don't seem to have done much of anything other than cost you money and make you feel like a loser. Not to make excuses, but the prolonged pandemic didn't help any.

Every morning when you go your closet and survey your options, it seems like you have fewer and fewer presentable outfits to wear. You have way too many cute dresses and pants that you wore routinely that now fit like sausage casings. You banish them from your sight so you don't start the day humiliating yourself by trying to squeeze into them only to immediately wriggle out of them. Pretty soon you may be down to a single pair of black slacks with a shirt and a long sweater that covers most of your sins. Not a good way to start the day on a positive note.

Last week you went in for your annual check-up and your blood work revealed an A1C level of 6.4%, which your physician advised you is in the high pre-diabetic range, bordering on full blown diabetes. OK then – maybe this is the to "Come-to-Jesus" moment you've needed. It's finally time to acknowledge that you've earned the right to pay attention to yourself and your health.

Are You Ready to Change Your Eating Habits?

One of the models that we wellness coaches learn is The Transtheoretical Model of the stages of change. It sounds very highfalutin, but it describes something important in terms of weight loss. The basic concept is that the decision to start getting serious about eating healthy foods in reasonable portions is not made lightly in today's food-focused environment.

Typically, we need to cycle through any number of quick weight loss diets before we finally decide that the only way to get the weight to stay away is to start eating healthy foods and to lose the fat at a slow pace.

The reason we resist this reality so vehemently is that we know it will involve hard work and some discomfort and that it will be a forever thing. We dread having to give up our most beloved friends – those favorite indulgent and snacky foods. We rely on them for comfort and convenience and the thought of weaning away from them and having to "be good" can seem like a bridge too far.

This book is intended to teach you how to assess whether or not you are ready to hit the healthy living trail. While the TM Model is a useful tool, we can use less technical, academic-sounding words in place of the more scholarly terms used by the model.

TM names the various stages as follows:
- Precontemplation
- Contemplation
- Preparation
- Action
- Maintenance
- Termination

I've come up with these more user-friendly terms:
- I'm Just Not Ready Yet

- I'm Starting to Think About it
- I'm Ready to Get Started
- I'm Doing it
- I Think I've Got This
- I Finally Have a Healthy Relationship with Food

This chapter deals with the first two phases of readiness to change.

THE "I'M JUST NOT READY YET" STAGE

In the "I'm Just Not Ready Yet" stage, you don't feel ready to make any changes in the foreseeable future. You're still telling yourself that everything is fine the way it is. But you do have a fairly persistent feeling that at some point you'll have to start working on your weight.

You can't deny the fact that some people eat a much healthier diet than you. You don't plan, so you eat what you enjoy and what is convenient. It works for you. You have a very busy life and no time to think about food. You don't really believe that the food you eat might be adversely affecting your health. You're just annoyed that every year you put on a few more pounds and it's starting to get out of control.

You have your aches and pains and sometimes feel like a slug, but doesn't everyone? Your friends complain about their ailments all the time, so it must be perfectly normal. So why bother making any changes?

THE "I'M STARTING TO THINK ABOUT IT" STAGE

The "I'm Starting to Think About it" stage is the phase that happens when you can actually envision making some changes to improve your health. You're thinking that you may just get started in the next six months.

You accept the fact that some of your habits are not serving you well and that you might reap some worthwhile health benefits if you start addressing the weaknesses in your diet that are only exacerbated with time.

Although the pull of maintaining your current behaviors is mighty strong, the urge to clean up your act is starting to give it a run for its money. You're still tethered to the fence, not feeling ready to make a move quite yet, but engaged in deep contemplation.

What Triggers Might Get You Started?

When you're vacillating between waiting until later (whenever that is) and taking the first step, a trigger is often required to get you to commit to doing the hard work of changing your health behaviors.

Sometimes you just don't know if you're ready to start making changes. I've had some clients who thought they were ready only to realize later that it was more of a pipe dream than an executable aspiration. To avoid making a false start and beating yourself up for failing, review these possible triggers and find out where you are in terms of your readiness to change.

> **Review each category of triggers below and decide whether you are in the "I'm Just Not Ready Yet," or the "I'm Thinking About it" stage.**

1. Your Blood Work Reveals Bad News

Learning that you have a medical condition like diabetes or high blood pressure is one of the most common triggers for beginning a weight loss program. A medical scare can be a "Come-to-Jesus" moment if you let it sink in and associate the cause with your poor lifestyle habits.

But many people "don't want to know," so they avoid going in for an annual physical and having a blood panel run. They rationalize that if they don't know that something is wrong or don't have an official diagnosis, they won't have to think about it or get it treated.

Many people tell themselves they don't have time to go see the doctor and since they feel fine, there's no reason to waste time waiting at their physician's office or having blood drawn to run a battery of useless tests.

Getting blood test results that show you are headed in the wrong direction can be a trigger for healthy lifestyle change.

> **Alarming medical news can be a trigger for healthy lifestyle change. Review the two stages below and see if you fall into either one.**

I'M JUST NOT READY YET

- I realize I need to get my blood work done, but I'm way too busy right now.
- I really don't think I need to go see my doctor this year because I'm feeling pretty good.
- I think doing blood work is probably going to be a waste of time since I feel fine.
- I just dread needles and can't even entertain the thought of getting blood drawn.
- I don't want to get a diagnosis of a health condition because I'm not ready to make any changes right now.

Does your thinking match this stage? Yes _____ No _____

I'M STARTING TO THINK ABOUT IT

- I've decided that I'm going to make an appointment with my doctor sometime soon.
- I'm going to go see my doctor and get a full workup as soon as work calms down in the next few months.
- I talked to a close friend who was recently diagnosed with cancer and I made a commitment to myself to go get my blood work done in the next few months.
- I promised my spouse that I'd make an appointment with my doctor to get a workup and I always keep my promises.
- I'm starting to obsess about my health going downhill and I've decided I need to go get a complete physical so I can stop worrying.

Or does your thinking match this stage? Yes _____ No _____

2. Decide You Need to Be a Role Model

Has it ever dawned on you that you're a role model for others, maybe your children, yet your behavior isn't exactly what you want them to emulate? Have you ever told your kids not to eat too many sweets and then been caught contradicting your own advice? At some point many parents vow to clean up their eating habits because they see their kids going down the same unhealthy eating path they've been traveling.

Change is hard. It's so much easier to hope that if you just say the right things, you won't be put to the test of practicing what you're preaching. The harsh truth is that children imitate their parents' behaviors and what you say to them amounts to "blah, blah, blah," unless you are demonstrating the eating habits you prescribe.

Something will trigger the realization that it's time to walk the walk, and not just talk the talk. You may realize that your children are starting to get a bit pudgy because of what they eat at home. Or you realize that social media is making your kids hypersensitive to weight issues when they start peppering you with questions about the family's eating habits and expressing anxiety about the prospect of being shunned because they don't have Instagram-worthy bodies. Other times, the urge to be a better role model is borne out of watching your own parents' health decline as a result of a lifetime of unhealthy eating habits, and making the decision to head in a much different direction toward a healthier old age.

> **Deciding that it's important for you to be a good role model can be a trigger for healthy lifestyle change. Review the two stages below and see if you fall into either one.**

How to Show Food Who's Boss

I'M JUST NOT READY YET

- I worry that my kids will develop my bad eating habits, but I'm not ready to change them right now.
- I'm concerned that I'm a bad Mom because I keep feeding my kids at the drive-thru, but I just don't have time to cook.
- I just had a baby and keep seeing all these overweight young kids, which makes me think that I'll need to start eating healthier eventually.
- I suspect that at some point I'll have to start practicing what I'm preaching because last night my daughter caught me inhaling that pint of ice cream right after I'd told her not to eat it.
- I wasn't exactly a paragon of healthy eating for my kids but maybe by the time my grandkids arrive I can do better.

Does your thinking match this stage? Yes ____ No ____

I'M STARTING TO THINK ABOUT IT

- I realize I need to start cleaning up my act soon since my kids are already getting a bit chubby.
- I know I need to seriously think about changing my eating habits because my daughter came home crying after some bullies at school called her "tubby."
- I read a book that talked about how kids model their parents' bad behavior even if they mouth good advice. I'm starting to realize I should actually model the advice I espouse.
- I know I need to change my eating habits because my daughter looks at social media all the time and is asking me all kinds of questions about our unhealthy diet.
- My husband got diagnosed with Type 2 diabetes, so I need to start cooking cleaner to help both of us lose weight.

Or does your thinking match this stage? Yes ____ No ____

3. You've Become Tired of Dragging Yourself Through the Day

Do you feel like you're dragging yourself through the day? Do you start out feeling less than energetic and become downright lethargic by noon? Do you fuel yourself with energy drinks or coffee just to keep your eyes open and your brain semi-functional?

If you're young, you may attribute your sluggishness to sleep deprivation or stress, whereas if you're over 40, you reflexively explain lethargy with that handy "I'm not as young as I used to be," excuse. We women like to place the blame for any health deficit on those ever-fluctuating hormones or to pin our hopes on our thyroid gland being out of whack. We'd like to avoid identifying the real culprits: lack of exercise, an unhealthy diet, and dragging extra weight around.

Finally deciding that you deserve a better life that includes waking up every morning feeling energetic and upbeat can be a good trigger for healthy lifestyle change.

> **Feeling tired and sluggish can be a trigger for healthy lifestyle change. Review the two stages below and see if you fall into either one.**

I'M JUST NOT READY YET

- I feel like I'm dragging myself around all the time, which I guess is just part of getting older.
- I know my doctor told me that if I lost some weight I'd have more energy, but I doubt it.
- I'm not sure why I feel so tired all the time, but it's probably just because my rebellious teenagers are stressing me out.
- I've felt like a total slug ever since I hit menopause, which is really a drag, but there's nothing I can do about that.
- I keep reading that your lifestyle choices make a difference in how you age, but I think it's all genetic.

Does your thinking match this stage? Yes ____ No ____

I'M STARTING TO THINK ABOUT IT

- I'm starting to see that there's a definite connection between feeling perpetually exhausted and the fact that I'm dragging around 40 lbs. of extra weight.
- I realize that it's probably about time to start emulating my healthy-eating college roommate who rivals the Energizer bunny™.
- I'm getting sick and tired of feeling sick and tired and am seriously considering hiring a Nutritionist within the next 6 months.
- I watched a YouTube video of Ernestine Shepard, an amazing 80-year-old female body builder, that convinced me it's not too late to start living a healthier life.
- I know I can't keep eating restaurant-prepared meals if I want to be healthy in my old age. I need to pivot to a healthier lifestyle before I start juggling a dozen prescription medications.

Or does your thinking match this stage? Yes ____ No ____

4. You See a Picture of Yourself and Hate the Way You Look

Many of my clients mention to me that one of the reasons they decided to seek out the assistance of a Nutritionist is that they were forced to look at themselves in a photo taken at a wedding or a family gathering. Despite wearing dark clothing in an effort to minimize their size, and their attempts to hide in the back, away from the camera, they're forced to see how they look and they hate what they see.

You can avoid looking in the mirror and try to camouflage the weight gain with forgiving baggy clothing, but at some point, you'll be forced to face reality and see what you really look like and it will have an impact. You may feel embarrassed or even shocked. Once you see the image, it's hard to erase it from your mind. Even if you immediately trash it from your phone, it's hard to deny the obvious any longer.

> **Seeing a picture of yourself and hating the way you look can be a trigger for healthy lifestyle change. Review the two stages below and see if you fall into either one.**

I'M JUST NOT READY YET

- I make up excuses to opt out of photo opportunities because I'm just not ready to see what I look like yet.
- I don't think I look that bad in photos but I'm not ready to test my theory.
- I refuse to look at pictures of myself at my current weight because I know I'll hate myself.
- I tell myself that the camera adds 10 pounds, so I'm still OK at my current weight.
- I retreat to the back row and hide if I get goaded into participating in a group photo.

Does your thinking match this stage? Yes _____ No _____

I'M STARTING TO THINK ABOUT IT

- I'm thinking that maybe I should diet before my sister's wedding so when I look at the pictures, I won't hate myself too much and it might even motivate me to change.
- I had a fleeting thought that I should finally take a look at the pictures my husband took on our Hawaii vacation last summer and see how bad I look.
- I almost asked my girlfriend to take a full body picture of me so I could see how fat I look.
- I've heard the expression "pictures don't lie," so maybe I need to compare some older pictures with the new ones and admit that I've gained quite a bit of weight.

Or does your thinking match this stage? Yes _____ No _____

5. Decide It's Finally Time to Pay Attention to Yourself

Many of my clients come to me after realizing that they've been neglecting their health for many years and finally deciding that it's the right time in their lives to pay some attention to themselves. Often mothers are so other-directed that they neglect their own health. They send their kids to school after feeding them a healthy breakfast and packing a nutritious lunch, but wait until noon, when they're starving, to eat something. They drive their kids to school, sports practice, and attend every event where they often end up eating whatever is available, which is usually unhealthy.

Often, around the time that our kids are going off to college or we're nearing retirement, we start to reflect on the time we have left. We want to make the best of it by taking off some weight so we'll have the energy to enjoy active lives or play with our grand kids.

> **Making the decision that you deserve to devote time to taking care of yourself can be a trigger for healthy lifestyle change. Review the two stages below and see if you fall into either one.**

I'M JUST NOT READY YET

- I know I've put on some weight but I don't have time to deal with it right now.
- I really need to start taking care of myself now that I've been diagnosed as pre-diabetic, but I just have too much going on right now.
- I know I need to start eating a healthier diet but that'll have to wait until I retire.
- I try to eat healthier but I can't seem to stay focused for any sustained period of time, so I guess it doesn't matter enough to me.
- I've vowed several times to buckle down and get the weight off, but I can't seem to get started because I have no idea what to do.

Does your thinking match this stage? Yes ____ No ____

I'M STARTING TO THINK ABOUT IT

- I'm retiring at the end of the year and I intend to hire a Nutritionist at that time.
- I know I need to take some weight off soon because I was playing with my grandkids and struggled for several minutes just to get up off the floor.
- I'm getting really worried about having to take so much medication and I know I can get off at least some of it if I start paying attention to my health.
- I see that my parents are not aging well and I need to stop following in their footsteps.
- I've raised three kids and they've all left the nest so now it's "me time."

Or does your thinking match this stage? Yes ____ No ____

6. Admit that Yo-Yo Dieting Doesn't Work

Almost everyone who wants to lose weight cycles through a series of quick weight loss diets. They starve themselves and lose some weight but then invariably suffer the disappointment of seeing it slowly creep back on like a boomerang. There are the ever-popular old standbys —Weight Watchers®, Lindora®, and Nutrisystem®. And then there are the trendy diets like Keto, Paleo, and Intermittent Fasting. All of these diets are based on calorie deprivation, so if you follow their strictures, you get the initial gratification of seeing the scale go in the preferable direction.

But the downfall of all of these diets is that at some point, you get tired of all the rules and restrictions and just give up. Once that happens, the weight starts reappearing, often with a few extra pounds that pile on as you reward yourself for exerting so much effort in your failed attempt to lose weight.

How many diets do you need to cycle through before you finally face the reality that you need to change your eating habits?

> **Admitting that yo-yo dieting doesn't work in the long term can be a trigger for healthy lifestyle change. Review the two stages below and see if you fall into either one.**

I'M JUST NOT READY YET

- I know the last three diets didn't work but I've heard great things about Keto, and my girlfriend swears by it since she lost 30 lbs. just by cutting out carbs.
- I'm really tired of losing and regaining weight, but I know it's my own fault and I'll try harder this time.
- I just have to stay focused and exert more willpower. I know I can lose the weight with Intermittent Fasting.
- I'll tackle losing the weight when I feel confident that I'll really stick to my diet.
- I just haven't found the diet that works for me, but I know it's out there.

Does your thinking match this stage? Yes _____ No _____

I'M STARTING TO THINK ABOUT IT

- I know trendy diets don't work for me and I need to try something different.
- I'm almost ready to give up on diets entirely and just start eating healthy.
- I realized today that no one I know who has lost weight fast has been able to keep it off.
- I think my doctor was right when she told me I need to change my eating habits to be healthy.
- I'm tired of feeling like a loser with diets. Maybe it's just time to change my relationship with food.

Or does your thinking match this stage? Yes _____ No _____

7. You'd Like to Be Able to Play with Your Grand Kids on the Floor

You may be at the stage in life where your two kids are finally both married off and you have your fingers crossed that being a grandma is on the horizon soon. You envision yourself as the fun grandma that your grand kids love to visit because you get down on the floor with them and play. The only part of the scenario that has you a bit worried is the getting up part. Last week you were arranging some china in a low cabinet and ended up sitting on the floor. When you tried to stand up you had to try three times before you struggled to your feet. You're embarrassed to admit that you were tempted to Google "how to get up off the floor."

You're not old enough to be a fat old lady who just sits on the couch and doesn't enjoy her grand kids and their boundless energy.

> **The desire to be able to play with your grand kids can be a trigger for healthy lifestyle change. Review the two stages below and see if you fall into either one.**

I'M JUST NOT READY YET

- I know my first grandchild is on the way in a few months and I probably won't be able to chase after her when she's a toddler.
- I've tried to play with my nieces on the floor, but I won't try that again because I had a hard time getting up.
- At my age, I have to grab onto a chair to get up off the floor, but that's just the way it is as you get older.
- I realize I need to lose some weight before the grand babies come, but I'm just not up to it at the moment.
- I'll just play with my grandkids on the couch or at the table because getting down on the floor isn't something I can do any more.

Does your thinking match this stage? Yes _____ No _____

I'M STARTING TO THINK ABOUT IT

- I started a new diet this week to get some weight off so I can move better, but I'm not sure I can stick with it.
- I want to be a more fun grandma, but I also love to eat out, and that puts on the pounds.
- I feel exhausted by my grandkids and I know if I get some weight off, it would help.
- I find myself making up excuses when my daughter asks me to babysit and I feel terrible about that.
- I don't like sitting on the couch and not playing with my grandkids, and I know my weight is the culprit.

Or does your thinking match this stage? Yes _____ No _____

8. You Want to Travel and Be Able to Walk

Perhaps you've dreamed of traveling the world when you retire or maybe you've just always had the travel bug. Either way, being mobile is pretty critical to an enjoyable experience. When you're carrying around the equivalent of a heavy sack of potatoes or a 50 lb. bag of rice, sightseeing on foot can be more like a visit to the dentist than a sojourn in paradise.

You know that if you don't have to worry about your aching knees, you'll be able to delight in the wonders of nature rather than praying that somehow, you'll be able to make it back to the trail head. It's hard to even envision a beach vacation, or imagine yourself poolside with a piña colada.

> **Wanting to get on a plane and explore the world can sometimes be a trigger for healthy lifestyle change. Review the two stages below and see if you fall into either one.**

I'M JUST NOT READY YET

- I want to travel the world but in my present state I'm just not ready to book any fun forays to exotic locales.
- I don't want to repeat the exhausting experience of walking all over Rome in excruciating pain.
- I love cruising but I need to be in shape for the day excursions or I'll be totally bored.
- I deserve a relaxing beach vacation but I'm embarrassed to be seen at my current weight unless I'm covered head to toe.
- No more hiking trips for me. Last time, I had to sit and rest so many times my friends lost patience and didn't invite me the next day.

Does your thinking match this stage? Yes _____ No _____

I'M STARTING TO THINK ABOUT IT

- I'm going to retire soon so I'm starting to think about how to improve my health so I can enjoy the retirement I've worked so hard to earn.
- I know I need to lose weight to travel, but I'm not sure I'm quite ready to give up my chips and ice cream.
- I feel the pressure of my non-refundable trip to Southeast Asia coming up, so I'd better lose some weight because I know we'll be walking a lot.
- I long to lounge around the pool luxuriating in the island breezes of Hawaii, but I know I'll enjoy it more if I lose some weight.

Or does your thinking match this stage? Yes _____ No _____

9. You Don't Want a Miserable Old Age with Chronic Diseases

When my career was focused on the baby boomer generation, I came up with this slogan to illustrate my ideal aging trajectory: "Healthy, healthy, healthy, healthy, dead." My intent was to get a laugh while promoting the goal of avoiding a painful, unsatisfying old age.

We're living longer and no one wants to give themselves a miserable old age struggling with chronic illness managed by poly-pharmacy. Most drugs have nasty side effects and treat only the symptoms of the ailment.

Sometimes we observe our parents or friends who are going down that path and we start worrying that we might be headed in that same direction, just a few beats behind. We start thinking about the fact that if we keep living the way we have been, we're likely going to be in feeble health far too soon.

> The prospect of a painful, dreary old age can be a trigger for healthy lifestyle change. Review the two stages below and see if you fall into either one.

I'M JUST NOT READY YET

- I've been feeling lousy since I went through menopause. I guess that's just a normal part of the aging process.
- I have less energy every year and it's probably because I eat an atrocious diet. But changing my habits now is impossible.
- I'm now taking diabetes meds and I know my unhealthy lifestyle is the reason. Thank God for modern medicine.
- I fondly recall my younger days when I felt healthy and energetic and I'd love to get back there, but I'm not up to exerting the effort.

Does your thinking match this stage? Yes _____ No _____

I'M STARTING TO THINK ABOUT IT

- I'm starting to think that the longer I wait to clean up my eating habits, the worse things are likely to be, so maybe I should get started sooner rather than later.
- I'm getting worried about being on so many meds. I'd better start eating healthier.
- I know I need to change my eating habits or I won't be cruising into a happy old age.
- I'm really getting worried about getting older with a laundry list of nagging aches and pains that prevent me from doing what I want.
- I know I should change my habits before I get any older, but I also wonder if it's already too late.

Or does your thinking match this stage? Yes _____ No _____

10. It's Time to Get Off Those Medications

Three-quarters of U.S. adults age 50 and over are on medication, filling as many as 13 different prescriptions every year. But drugs are not a free ride. They all have potential side effects and there's the complex issue of drug interactions. In addition to the physician prescribed meds, about 70% of adults take over-the-counter supplements, which are not regulated by the FDA and may, in some cases, be dangerous.

Most of the clients who come to me are already taking meds for high blood pressure, high cholesterol, or diabetes. Some are motivated toward change immediately, and others take the drugs for several years before they decide that a better answer is to clean up their eating habits.

> **A desire to live drug free can be a trigger for healthy lifestyle change. Review the two stages below and see if you fall into either one.**

I'M JUST NOT READY YET

- I'm getting tired of the side effects of all the medications I'm on, but such is life.
- I hate taking all these drugs, but at least I'm not worried about having a heart attack.
- I yearn for my younger days when I was full of energy and not living on drugs to get me through the day, but those days are long gone.
- I have to take a handful of pills just to face the day without worrying about stroking out. I hate that, but it is what it is.
- I'm very jealous of my sister who doesn't take any drugs. I'm now up to eight every day. I guess we didn't inherit the same genes.

Does your thinking match this stage? Yes _____ No _____

I'M STARTING TO THINK ABOUT IT

- I wonder if losing weight might help me get off some of my prescription meds.
- I'm starting to seriously think about starting to eat healthy so I can lose the weight that's causing me to need all these drugs.
- I'm so fed up with the permanently upset stomach caused by my cholesterol and high blood pressure medications and I need to do something to get off them.
- I know I need to make a drastic lifestyle change if I don't want to be a prescription drug junkie forever.
- I'm almost ready to follow my husband and start eating healthy so I can get off some of my meds like my husband did.

Or does your thinking match this stage? Yes _____ No _____

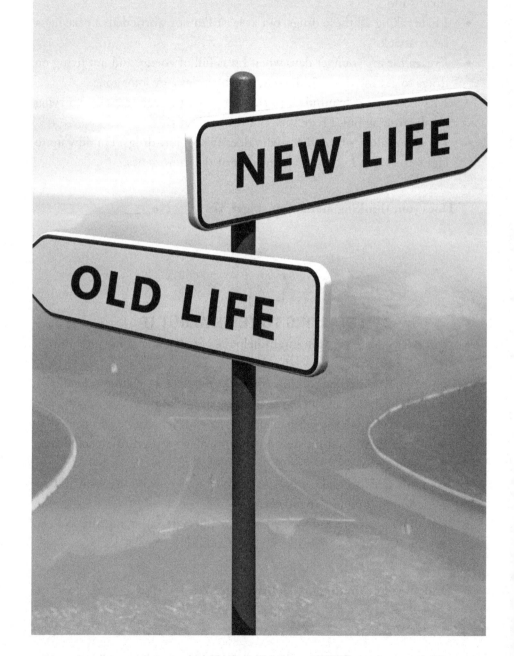

3

How Brain Change Works on Habits

Does This Sound Familiar?

If you've reached the preparation stage, you feel like "I'm ready to get started." You've accepted the fact that you really do have to change your eating habits or you're doomed to a miserable old age. You're thinking that within the next month you can get your head around starting to think about making some changes.

You're reluctant to do a cartwheel into the deep end of the pool only to decide that the water is far too cold, so that you shy away for a few more years. This time you try something radically different. You surprise yourself by just dipping your toe in the water. Your toe feels like it has frostbite, but because you're getting acclimated to the change, it feels less traumatic and more achievable.

In the action stage you feel like "I'm all in. I'm doing it!" For the first time in your life, you've decided to bite the bullet and learn how to cope with all the temptations around you instead of following a prescribed diet that obviates the need to ever figure that out. You've tried allowing diet gurus to tell you what to eat so many times, and you're finally getting comfortable with the notion of making a steady, sustained effort to get healthy. Your baby steps are accumulating to the point that you actually feel more energetic and can start to see some results. Even though the changes feel uncomfortable, you stay motivated to keep moving down the healthy path. It feels challenging yet doable.

If this resonates with your current attitude about losing weight, then you are ready to begin. One important criteria of success is to first understand how behavior change works so that you begin with realistic expectations.

1. Identify Habits You're Ready to Change

The first step in the long-delayed spring cleaning of your body is to take a breath and rein yourself in a bit. Your first inclination after making this belated decision to buckle down and get to the root of the problem — your eating habits — is to go full-bore into dieting mode and try to starve off the pounds. This should not come as a surprise, as this is the only mode you've ever practiced when you've been serious about losing weight.

The type of traditional diets you've used in the past have a laundry list of rules and provide strict weight loss guidelines, which no one can live with for an extended period of time. Going on a diet has always required a titanic, abrupt change in your lifestyle. You've gone along with the program because you've been desperate.

But at some point, you yearn for normalcy. You give up the extreme mandates of the diet because they clash with your real life which includes enjoying food and social activities. For example, your 600-calorie day of Intermittent Fasting happens to coincide with the day you're going out to celebrate your husband's birthday. Diet over. Or you're on Keto and your colleague's going-away dinner is at Olive Garden™. You're already salivating thinking about the chicken alfredo and breadsticks. Game over.

Lifestyle change is an entirely different beast from any type of "diet" you've surrendered to in the past. In fact, it's a new way to think about your relationship with food and to achieve the feeling that you are in charge of what goes into your mouth. The concept of lifestyle change is to start to pay attention to your eating habits, and then to incrementally alter those habitual patterns with slow upgrades. Unlike your past efforts to lose weight, this behavior change happens in a relatively seamless way that fits into your current lifestyle.

How to Show Food Who's Boss

Bottom line: You're going to acquire new skills that will allow you to live in the real world. This will feel very different from the just-tell-me-what-to-eat diets that have worked initially and then failed you in the long run.

When you begin making permanent changes to your eating habits, you start to realize what you're up against. We live in a society that is nothing less than obsessed with food. Every place you look there is an abundance of edibles, most of them sorely lacking in healthy nutrition. The challenge of lifestyle change is to consistently make healthy choices despite the onslaught of junk food available everywhere you turn. Our food-focused world is very much at odds with a healthy diet. It features gigantic portions of heavily processed foods swimming in butter and oil and containing lab-concocted, taste-bud addicting proportions of salt, sugar, and fat.

Once you decide to change your ways, the next step is to be totally honest with yourself about which parts of your dietary habits you are actually ready to start improving. We all have crutches we're just not ready to give up; at least not immediately. It might be the chill-out glass of wine or two that you consume nightly. Or maybe it's your chocolate after dinner treats. That's OK. Leave them be. Don't try to fix everything that you think is broken in the first week. Doing so will stress you out, overwhelm you, and make you feel like quitting before you even get started.

Instead, identify two or three unhealthy habits that you've been itching to break for some time, but you haven't gotten around to facing. Then create some very small steps that get you moving towards that goalpost.

Examples of Small Steps Towards a Bigger Goal

Goal #1	Stop mindless junk-food snacking after dinner. Choose fruit after dinner on two nights instead of cookies. The other five nights, keep your cookies.
Goal #2	Stop getting grab-n-go every night because there's nothing to eat in the house. Do a meal plan so you have at least three meals planned for the week. The other nights, keep the carryout.
Goal #3	Avoid getting home from work starving. Bring a healthy snack to work, like an apple or a handful of nuts, that you can eat it on the way home and see if it makes you less tempted to scarf down the first thing you see when you cross the threshold.
Goal #4	Stop mindless Netflix munching. Instead of your usual chips, experiment once by substituting air popped popcorn spritzed with oil and spiced up.
Goal #5	Conquer your mid-afternoon pick-me-up. Twice next week, try eating a healthy snack that you brought from home instead of making your Starbucks™ run.

2. Don't Be Ashamed to Hire a Health Coach

Developing a healthy relationship with food is confoundingly difficult. It's a bit puzzling. No one shoves food into our mouths. We are in control of our jaw muscles. Yet, sticking to healthy foods and not overeating don't come easy. It's almost as if the jaw muscle has a mind of its own and we are not in charge. Very few of us can get through the day making conscious healthy food choices and avoiding empty calories and processed foods.

Why is that? I've identified two main culprits: (1) the food environment, and (2) using food to satisfy emotional needs.

The Food Environment

When I was growing up, which is before most of you readers were born, we ate what our mothers cooked. My mother may have been the world's worst chef, but she had no choice. A typical dinner consisted of mushy, salty, tasteless canned vegetables, a lump of bland mashed potatoes or rice, and some sort of inexpensive meat cooked to shoe leather consistency to ensure we were not exposed to salmonella. Only if I choked down all my veggies did I earn dessert. Overeating was never a temptation. I was overjoyed when Swanson® TV Dinners made their appearance in grocery stores and relieved my mother of trying to be a decent cook.

Drive-thrus were brand new and my family shunned them. Restaurants were not in the take-out business. Dining out in a restaurant was a once-a-year special treat. My parents did buy sweets but they were kept under lock and key and doled out only in small doses as rewards.

When I think back on my grade school and high school classmates, I realize that the overweight ones were few and far between. The food environment simply did not encourage the type of overeating it does today. Also, kids ran around outside and played, unlike today when they closet themselves in their rooms tethered to their tech toys.

Using Food to Satisfy Emotional Needs

The saturated food environment encourages us to use snack food as a way to meet our emotional needs. We've got plenty of food in the house, so it's easy to start snacking and then it just snowballs. It tastes great and it seems to do the trick in the moment. It's only later that we regret it and get bummed out by our behavior.

Chronic stress is one of the big drivers. Living in permanent flight-or-fight mode increases production of cortisol which then stimulates our appetites, particularly for sugary, salty, and fatty foods.

But it's not just stress that causes us to go for munchies. Medicating ourselves with food works for the full panoply of emotions. You may indulge in sweets or crunchy, salty snacks when you're bored, when you feel a need to reward yourself, when you're frustrated, when you finally get some "me time," or as a mindless accompaniment to binge watching Netflix.

There never seems to be a shortage of temptations on hand. Sometimes they jump off the shelves and into our carts as we navigate the grocery store aisles, or we bake cookies for a colleague's birthday party and stash a few extras in the kitchen cupboard. See's Candies® or tempting leftovers from social gatherings are typically sitting around the house. If not, DoorDash™ or one of the other delivery services will be happy to bring you any treat you want in an hour or less.

Why You Need a Health Coach

I'm confident that I have convinced you that changing your health habits will feel like fighting a rip current. The pull of ingrained habits is powerful, and we act on those patterns on a semi-automatic basis without even having to make a conscious decision. Endeavoring to eat healthy in today's society is so formidable that it is nearly impossible make the transition without a health coach.

Many people believe they can win this battle on their own and start with a burst of enthusiasm and a focused determination. "This time I'm serious and I'm going to get the weight off!" A likely choice these days is to opt to go Keto since you probably know several people who've lost weight on that diet.

Since Keto is a bit tricky, you start with a detailed meal plan and decide you're going to spend Sunday preparing a week's worth of healthy food. You're on point with the diet during the initial week, but the next Sunday, you just can't talk yourself into devoting the time and energy to meal planning and prepping, so you do a modified version of the diet on the fly. By week #3, you're too busy with social engagements and kids' soccer games and you can't even focus on sticking to such a rigorous diet. Even though you managed to bring your lunch, you find yourself saying yes to your co-worker's invitation to go to The Habit™. You're starving and feeling entitled to be bad, so you inhale your favorite Charburger Combo with fries. You do momentarily consider, and quickly reject, the lettuce wrap option. You feel bun deprived! Instead, you make a lame effort to ameliorate the damage by ordering a Diet Coke® instead of a regular.

You pay for your overindulgence for the rest of the day, feeling bloated and lethargic and more than a little displeased with yourself. You give up for the rest of the week and vow to start anew next Monday. But then the weekend turns out to be a social whirlwind and you start the week without much of anything in the house since you had no time to go grocery shopping.

You start to doubt your ability to go it alone on the weight loss journey. You also begin to question whether your choice of the Keto was the best option. You're starting to hear a lot of buzz about Intermittent Fasting. Maybe you should give that one a try.

Or maybe it's time to just admit that you don't know how to do this on your own. You have a girlfriend who hired a Nutritionist a few years ago, lost a significant amount of weight and seems to be keeping it off. Time to Google "Nutritionist."

3. Make Changes in Baby Steps

Most people have two diametrically opposed modes of eating. They are either on the "see-food" diet, which entails eating whatever makes them happy, or they are on a "diet." The latter involves strict rules about what they can and cannot eat and calorie limits to the point of feeling hungry most of the time.

Neither eating pattern is optimal. How about a middle ground, where you purposefully pause eating on autopilot and start paying attention to what you're eating? This is the beginning of the journey to healthy eating. It may lack the flash and flare of the latest trend in dieting, but it proves its pedigree when your weight stays consistent after you reach your goal. The reason is simple. You have finally developed a relationship with food which allows you to purposefully make good choices.

The problem with diet mode is that it's never sustainable. You'll only put up with starving yourself and eliminating your food groups for so long. For some period of time the scale will be your happy place, but then it will stall or you'll just decide you're tired of depriving yourself and go back to what you were eating pre-diet.

Let's say you were able to lose 15 lbs. on Keto and that was your goal. Now you're at the panicked stage where you worry it will all come back on after all that work. And lo and behold, it does. The only variable is how long it will take.

There are two reasons that the lost weight will find your gut or your backside again.

- A quick weight loss diet results in losing water weight and often lean muscle mass. The latter is particularly unfortunate because it will slow down your metabolism. The water weight will come back on once you resume eating some semblance of a normal diet.

- You will default to the see-food diet that sent you scrambling to lose weight in the first place because you didn't do anything to change that pattern.

Impatience is the way of the world today. We're used to instantaneous results in every facet of our lives. If a website takes more than 2-3 seconds to load, we click away and try another site. If my own website doesn't come up immediately, I panic and assume the worst — I've been hacked. Technology has ruined our ability to look at the road ahead and be satisfied when we are making steady progress in the right direction.

Slow and Steady Yields Results

It's so hard to go the tortoise and not the hare route today. But behavior doesn't turn on a dime. It takes a lot of repetition to form a habit, but once you do, it becomes second nature, feels very comfortable, and requires little or no thought to execute it.

To extricate yourself from a food habit you first have to acknowledge the behavior. For example, you may be in the habit of going to Taco Bell™ for lunch and ordering the Chicken Quesadilla Combo. You don't even think about whether it's healthy. It tastes good and you know it will be satisfying. It doesn't enter your mind to look at the menu and consider ordering something else. You're comfortable with your tried-and-true and you automatically order and eat it without having to engage in any cognitive thought process.

Let's say you want to change that habit. Your first instinct might be to go cold turkey and ban Taco Bell™ from your life. While it may sound like a reasonable approach, it almost always results in failure. Instead, set a goal to make a small change that's not so disconcerting. Maybe you could try just ordering a quesadilla and not having the taco. That's a baby step in the right direction.

4. Set Measurable Goals that Feel 75% Doable

Here's the way successful behavior change works. Start paying attention to your food habits, decide which ones are doing you a disservice, and set very specific goals that feel 75% achievable.

If you habitually go to Taco Bell™ for lunch and you want to change that pattern, your ultimate goal might be to pare it down to a once in a while treat. But don't do that immediately because you will be hating life. A reasonable first step would be to cut down the frequency to three times next week instead of five, and eat healthier foods the other days. Once you achieve that goal on a regular basis, then you move the goalpost a bit further down the field. Ultimately you may decide you don't' want to totally banish "Think Outside the Bun©" from your life. That's okay. It can stay in your food repertoire as an occasional treat.

Don't expect that the changes will stick after the 21-day mythical period of time. There is no scientific basis for that widely bandied-about number. In reality, how long it will take you to replace a bad habit with a better one, and have it feel comfortable, depends on a multitude of factors including how ready you were to change the behavior, the strength of your motivation, how quickly you find a tolerable substitution, and whether there's any social pressure involved.

Think of habit change in terms of a trail with switchbacks. Sometimes you get confused and double back, occasionally you lose focus and wander off the trail or take the wrong fork, but eventually, if you just keep moving ahead, you reach that beautiful waterfall.

5. Keep a Food Diary for Accountability

If you want to lose weight, tracking your food and drink intake is essential. In fact, people lose twice as much weight when they keep a food diary. I recommend the MyFitnessPal™ app to my clients because it allows diary sharing with friends. It means my clients know that I am watching them in between our weekly sessions. It ups the accountability quotient significantly.

Here are some persuasive reasons to track your intake:

- It will force you to learn portion sizes
- You will be forced to see your current eating habits
- It may deter you from overeating
- It will give you a reasonable calorie goal to focus on
- It will teach you how many calories are in restaurant prepared food
- It will help you identify your emotional eating
- It will teach you that you can eat too many calories of healthy food
- You can share it for extra accountability
- It has a deterrent effect on mindlessly eating junk food
- It prevents you from being in denial about what you ate

6. Focus on Food Quality More Than Calorie Intake

Don't make the mistake of focusing just on reducing calories as a weight loss technique. Eating healthy is more than calories-in-calories-out. And don't think your body doesn't care what you put in your mouth. Your body is not ignorant. It knows whether you ate healthy whole foods or junky, processed fast food. Whole foods will make you feel good. Junk food will make you feel lethargic, bloated, and sluggish.

Another reason to focus on food quality is to keep yourself full. When you eat processed foods, your body has a very easy time finishing the food processing. This is because most of the work was already done before you ate it. Your body will quickly absorb whatever meager nutrients it can find and then you'll be looking around for a snack because you're hungry again. Despite the shockingly high number of calories in the fast food, the meal won't keep you feeling full for very long.

But if you make healthier choices like fruits, vegetables, lean proteins, and other whole foods which haven't been adulterated with massive amounts of fat and sugar, you give your gastrointestinal system a significant amount of work to do to extract the nutrients and send the waste materials packing. While your body is doing its magic, you'll still feel full and you'll be burning calories in the process.

When you're trying to lose weight, it's helpful to be able to stay full for about four or five hours after each meal. That obviates the need to make food decisions all day. The less you focus on making food choices, the fewer opportunities your brain gets to go to nefarious places.

The key nutrient in terms of fullness is protein, and it needs to be consumed in reasonable amounts throughout the day or it will not be properly absorbed. Aim for about 20 to 30 grams of protein with each meal and you won't feel the need to scour the office or root through your cupboards for some candy or a bag of chips.

7. Work on Portion Control

Have you heard the term "portion distortion?" It refers to the fact that portions have ballooned in the last 20 years. Standard portions of many common foods, like bagels and pasta, have doubled in size. Twice the size translates into twice the calories.

To make matters worse on the healthy eating front, plate size has steadily increased from 8 inches to an average of 12 inches or more. Restaurant plates have been replaced with what we used to call serving dishes. It's become commonplace for dining establishments to tap into the "more for your money" mentality with "all you can eat" buffets, coupon deals, and Roman banquet-style extravagant brunches. The purpose of doling out gargantuan amounts of rich food is to keep customers happy. Diners who believe they have gotten their money's worth tend to become loyal customers.

Since we like to fill our plates and finish every last morsel, these trends lead us to unwittingly consume the amount of food that an Olympic athlete might need to prepare for competition. Meanwhile, most of us burn a lot fewer calories than our grandparents did when jobs were physically demanding. Desk jockeys don't need much food for their somnambulant bodies.

There is an important distinction to be made between portion sizes (the amount in the package or on the plate) and USDA serving sizes. They describe quite different amounts of food. As an example, a serving size of fish, chicken, or steak is the size of your palm or a deck of cards. No restaurant would dare to serve such a minute portion and risk disgruntled diners who might post a negative Yelp review and never return.

I recently bought a 9-1/2 inch size dinner plate as a visual illustration for my clients. I also filled the plate with portions of different foods according to USDA recommendations, which include covering half the plate with low calorie, nutritious vegetables. My exemplar is nothing like what most people are eating and that's the point I'm trying to demonstrate.

8. Ban the Scale

I hate the scale. I don't equivocate on this topic unless the client, against my advice, braves the scale and happens to be pleased with the number. My advice to all of my clients is NOT to use the scale to track their weight loss.

The scale is a frightfully inaccurate mechanism when used to measure the intentionally slow weight loss achieved through lifestyle changes. It jumps up and down like a Chihuahua who needs to go outside after being closeted in a New York efficiency apartment. I've monitored my daily weight with the scale and found that it routinely fluctuates by about ½ to 1 pound up or down from day to day.

Here are just some of the day-to-day variations that can affect the number on the scale:

- Water retention from sodium or carbohydrates
- Not weighing yourself first thing in the morning before consuming food or drink
- No bowel movement
- Chronic stress
- Muscles repairing themselves after exercise
- Certain medications
- Hormonal fluctuations
- Unprocessed alcohol
- Illness
- Not placing the scale on a hard surface

Because the scale is demotivating more often than not, I steer my clients away from using it as their primary weight loss tracker. I try to convince them to avoid it by posing the question as to whether anyone, on first meeting, has ever asked them for their weight. The answer is a puzzled, sheepish "no." Pay attention to your body and how your clothes fit. Those indicators tell the tale and don't vacillate day-to-day.

9. Measure Progress with Body Changes

If the scale is not the answer to weight loss tracking, what tool works better?

The body tells the tale. That seems pretty obvious. When you're losing weight, your body is changing. We are so conditioned to treating the scale as the indisputable Weight Oracle, that even though I tell my clients that I wish this unreliable and inaccurate device had never been invented, they still can't resist stepping on. While it is fairly reliable on a long-term basis, on a daily or weekly basis, it's not the least bit credible.

Yet most of my clients succumb to its siren call despite my warnings that more often than not, they will come away demotivated and depressed. Perhaps the culprit is 60 years of effective marketing by Weight Watchers®.

Instead, I coach my clients to focus on eating a healthier diet first and foremost, and to treat their weight loss as a "happy by-product" of getting healthier. Pay attention to the changes healthy eating makes in your body. For most people, the first noticeable effect is that their energy level improves. Many people also have fewer gastrointestinal issues and enjoy deeper sleep. They notice that they lose those extra chins that have accumulated over the years and that their faces acquire more definition. Then they try on a pair of old jeans and find that they are able to zip them all the way up and button them. At this point no one can deny that the fat is disappearing.

10. Find the Balance That Allows You to Have a Normal Social Life

If you're going to lose weight and actually prevent it from creeping back on, there is no short-cut to doing it in a way that forces you to learn how to live in the real world, which includes attending social events, going on vacation, and enjoying restaurant dining.

The trendy diets like Keto and Intermittent Fasting may help you ditch some water weight and lean muscle mass, but at some point, everyone says "enough already!" and resumes normal eating. That's when the weight gets on a fast track to reapply itself wherever you'd least like to see it show up. And your penalty after exerting all that self-control is a few extra pounds resulting from slowing down your metabolism while you were starving yourself.

The irony of the miracle weight loss diets is that in the long run, you waste a lot of time, and sometimes take a serious hit to your bank account, because you get into the vicious cycle of losing and regaining. Even worse, there is emerging research showing that yo-yo dieting takes a toll on your health including increasing your risk of heart problems.

Lifestyle change certainly goes against the grain in our immediate-gratification society where all results must be instantaneous and effortless or we become extremely impatient and annoyed. But the faster the weight disappears, the quicker it reappears. Ironically, slow turns out to be faster.

The other major after-effect of this speedy weight loss and regain syndrome is that it takes a toll on your self-confidence. It leads you to believe that you're incapable of ever losing weight and looking good again. You start to think that you are doomed to a life of baggy dark clothing and hiding from mirrors and cameras. Understand that you did not fail, the diets failed you.

So go find some patience somewhere and lose weight in a way that allows you to have a normal, happy life; not one in which you are starving yourself all day and obsessing about food. Our relationship with food is out of balance and we need to find a new one that works for us despite the fact that unhealthy food beckons 24/7.

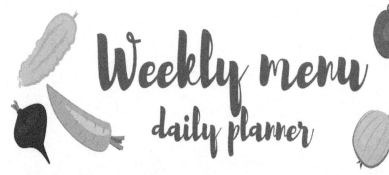

Weekly menu
daily planner

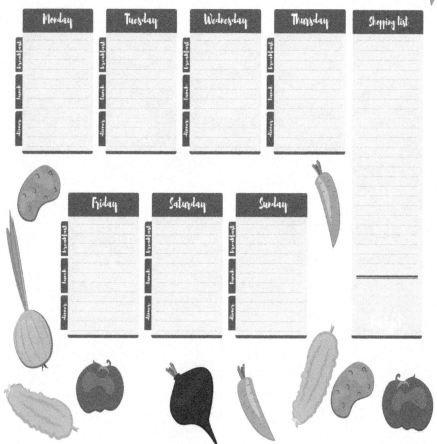

Monday	Tuesday	Wednesday	Thursday	Shopping list
breakfast	breakfast	breakfast	breakfast	
lunch	lunch	lunch	lunch	
dinner	dinner	dinner	dinner	

Friday	Saturday	Sunday
breakfast	breakfast	breakfast
lunch	lunch	lunch
dinner	dinner	dinner

4

How to Stay Motivated Through the Changes

Does This Sound Familiar?

You're about a month into your healthy eating program. You've lost 8 pounds so far, which is good, but you feel like the weight is coming off incredibly slowly. You keep thinking about when you did Keto and lost 15 lbs. in the same amount of time. Reality check: You craved carbs the whole time, couldn't eat out with your friends, and gained it all back.

Still, your resolve is wavering. You have 22 more pounds to lose and that's going to take quite a few more months. You know that meal planning and prep are the keys, but you're getting tired of devoting so much time to that task every weekend. Summer is coming, which means a vacation in San Francisco and then a visit to Disneyland with extended family. You're dying to try the cutting-edge restaurants everyone talks about in the Bay Area and you know there are lots of snacky temptations at theme parks.

You start to try to justify "taking a break" during the 10-day vacation, but you're afraid you'll undermine your pitifully meager progress and go into a deep depression. Eating at home where you have control over the food offerings now feels doable, but traveling presents daunting and unpredictable situations. It

---

seems like curtailing your usual "I'm on vacation and all bets are off" mentality may be beyond your bandwidth. You're not at all confident you're up to the task.

You ultimately decide not to stress out over it and to just go with the flow. You tell yourself if you succeed in not packing on more pounds during your time away, you'll be pretty happy with yourself.

When you get home, you dread the scale weigh-in so you postpone it for a few weeks during which you don't feel like being very diligent and haven't really gotten out of vacation mode. The Monday you finally get on the scale is not a good day.

Introduction

Most people begin their weight loss efforts like an inexperienced runner doing her first 10K race. When the starting gun sounds, you take off like a Thoroughbred at the Kentucky Derby. After a few miles you're huffing and puffing and your legs feel like rubber. You wonder if you'll even make it to the finish line. What you learn is that you'll achieve a better result if you pull back the reins a bit at the beginning and focus on maintaining a steady, viable pace until you see the finish line. Then you can go like a racehorse.

Somehow this concept proves incredibly difficult for us to apply to weight loss. When we finally decide it's time to lose weight and develop the coping skills we need in our food-centric environment, we want instantaneous results. We are an impatient lot. We conveniently forget that the weight crept on slowly pound by pound. We don't pay much attention to the accumulation. We just choose denial for as long as possible. Then one day we're tired of being overweight and decide to act. Then we want the fat to dissolve like butter in a hot pan. But the reality is that it comes off the same way, slowly but surely. Trying to accelerate the process with a quick weight loss diet just costs even more time, since we end up stuck in a frustrating lose/regain cycle.

Once you accept the long-haul view, the trick is to keep your eye on the ball and to consistently push forward. Along the way there will be many off-ramps and curves which lead back to your bad habits. Resisting each and every one of them is literally impossible. Aiming for perfection is the wrong goalpost. Just do the best you can and when you slip, forgive yourself and get back at it. That's the secret to learning to develop a healthy relationship with food.

10 Ways to Stay on Track

Despite all the opportunities that present themselves to get you off track and to go back to your poor eating habits, with patience and persistence you can stay on track.

1. Celebrate Small Achievements

THE MINDSET THAT GETS YOU OFF TRACK

You've lost 5 lbs. during your first month of healthy eating. While you're happy to ditch some fat, your clothes are not really fitting a lot better, the scale is down but only a little, and worst of all you still have 25 lbs. to go.

You start to think that this is too steep a hill to climb. You've been really good for a month, but you don't really have confidence that you can keep it up, and the rewards are just not materializing fast enough.

You're very tempted to just bag this healthy eating method and go back to Keto or try Intermittent Fasting to get the weight loss to speed up.

THE MINDSET THAT KEEPS YOU ON TRACK

To stay on track, you need to shift your mindset. Instead of focusing on how many pounds you still have to lose, set some short-term goals and celebrate each mini achievement. This technique has the added benefit of forcing you to think about how to reward yourself in ways that don't involve food.

You might decide to acknowledge your success every time you lose 10 lbs. or, better yet, when you fit back into your favorite jeans.

Some ideas for your celebration:

- Spend a day at the beach
- Go for a long hike with a friend
- Get a massage
- Get a manicure and/or a pedicure
- Enjoy a spa day
- Buy a small indulgence
- Go on a mini shopping spree
- Take a mini vacation
- Go to a concert

2. Focus on How Far You've Come

THE MINDSET THAT GETS YOU OFF TRACK

You've lost a few pounds but you're feeling discouraged because eating healthy is work and the weight seem to be coming off at a snail's pace. You've done lots of other diets where the scale went down a lot faster than it does with a lifestyle change program.

You're starting to lose momentum when you do the arithmetic and calculate how long it's going to take to get to your goal at your current rate. You still have a long road ahead and it doesn't seem to be getting any easier. In fact, you feel like you're so far from the finish line you can't even see it.

Then your thoughts take a turn for the worse and you end up telling yourself that "I'll always be overweight. I can't do this." Yet you also know that you need to get healthy for a laundry list of reasons. But your brain continues to bombard you with negative thoughts. You wonder, will I ever get there?

THE MINDSET THAT KEEPS YOU ON TRACK

To stay on track, you need to shift your mindset back to the starting line. Don't even think about that yellow tape right now.

Focus on where you started and take note of the many changes you've already made that show real progress. Then put your brain in the positive place of feeling good about the incremental improvements that have now become second nature.

Some positive mindset thoughts:
- You've decreased the amount of restaurant dining you do
- You've learned that you can assemble a healthy meal quickly without cooking from scratch
- You've decreased your portion sizes at meals and don't go back for seconds
- You've learned that frozen meals can be a life saver
- You're a lot more conscious of what you put in your mouth
- You've educated yourself on the number of calories in various foods
- You've learned to tolerate eating vegetables
- You've made your food environment less tempting

3. Take Pictures of Your Improving Physique Periodically

THE MINDSET THAT GETS YOU OFF TRACK

Even though you are losing weight you still look away as you walk by the hall mirror. You don't pose for selfies and avoid group photos if you can get away with it. Every picture you've seen of yourself since you gained all that weight has made you feel humiliated.

Instead, you stick with the mercurial scale and treat its electronic numbers like the Word of God. You ride the number waves and get depressed whenever it goes up ½ lb. You know it might go down the next day, but you let it ruin your day anyway.

THE MINDSET THAT KEEPS YOU ON TRACK

To stay on track, you need to shift your mindset away from total devotion to the scale. When you lose weight your body changes. The weight may not be coming off in the places where it annoys you the most, but it is coming off somewhere.

Keeping a photo diary is an easy way to chart your weight loss. Some of the weight loss apps even encourage you to do so. Most people see changes in their face first. Then all bets are off. Bodies are different. Some clients report that their back fat shrinks and many note changes in the size of their thighs. Unfortunately, most people want the belly fat to go away, and usually that is not the first area to shrink. But eventually it succumbs.

These visual results have an impact. A pictorial record is a lot more likely to lift you up than dealing with the scale as your measure of progress. As they say, pictures don't lie.

4. Tell Your Family and Friends That You're Trying to Get Healthier

THE MINDSET THAT GETS YOU OFF TRACK

You've tried so many diets and failed that this time, you decided not to say anything to anyone. You don't want to endure the skeptical looks or invite your family and friends to turn into the food police. You're sort of hedging your bets. This way, if you fail, at least no one knows about it but you.

But there is a downside to this choice. When you eat with your friends, they ask why you ordered a salad with a chicken breast on top and limited yourself to a single drink. Then you have to come up with some excuse on the fly. And you find it very hard to try to hold the line when your girlfriends are in party mode at your favorite restaurant and fully expect that you will overindulge right along with them as you always have. Your husband brings lots of chips and cookies into the house and resisting that temptation seems to require more willpower than you have in your reservoir at the end of a long day.

THE MINDSET THAT KEEPS YOU ON TRACK

To stay on track, it helps to create external accountability. The way to do this is to solicit support from other human beings. If you tell them that you're on a health journey, you will find that they will generally support you. Some might even admire your efforts or use you as a role model. That doesn't mean you need to shout it from the rooftops. Just select a few people who you trust to offer encouragement and perhaps hold you accountable when you ask them for help.

Behavior change is uncomfortable and old habits die hard. The process feels overwhelming at times and you will feel the pull of reverting to the patterns you followed for so many years. At these moments it can be extremely helpful to get support and gentle reminders.

5. If You Veer Off Track a Bit, Just Get Right Back On

THE MINDSET THAT GETS YOU OFF TRACK

You were doing so well, eating healthy and resisting tempting treats. You were even thinking "I've got this!" Then a curve ball came your way and you struck out big time.

You and your husband went to dinner with another couple who are not the healthiest eaters on the planet, and you broke your vow to only have one drink. They ordered another round for the table and it was too hard to resist.

You did well with the entrée. You abided by your plan to order the salmon dish and you asked for veggies instead of rice. You even remembered to order your To-Go box with your entrée and removed half of the food from your sight.

But then the waiter came by with the dessert menus and everyone wanted to indulge. You'd intended to pass on sweets, but you hadn't had crème brulee in so long you could taste it. Plus, the over-the-top recommendation by the waiter got your mouth watering. You were able to stop yourself before you ate the whole ramekin and quickly shoved it over to your husband who was happy to finish the rest.

On the drive home you started berating yourself for straying from your plan. You were so disappointed in yourself that you let your perspective spin out of control. You lectured yourself. You didn't need that extra drink and should have gotten a decaf coffee when everyone else was indulging in caloric desserts.

THE MINDSET THAT KEEPS YOU ON TRACK

To stay on track, you need to stop expecting perfection from yourself. This is a trait that I've struggled with most of my life so I can certainly empathize with my clients when they beat themselves up over not achieving 100% of the goals we set for the week.

Do not ever expect yourself to be perfect when you are trying to make changes to your diet. It is a process of trial and error, and failure is an expected and normal part of that process. Sometimes the goals turn out to be too aggressive, other times the situation is not as expected, and many times a lack of planning prevents you from being totally successful.

Instead of aiming for perfection and setting yourself up for disappointment and self-flagellation, go into the behavior change journey with a realistic attitude.

6. When You Totally Blow it, Practice Self-Compassion

THE MINDSET THAT GETS YOU OFF TRACK

You totally blew it today. It was Cinco de Mayo, you'd just suffered through a trying day at work, and were relishing a little time to relax. You were also feeling like you'd been deprived of any type of fun for over two years, and when you walked into your friend's house and saw the spread of food and drink, all resolve to "be good" immediately evaporated.

As soon as you got in the door someone put a Margarita in your hand, and you weren't about to refuse it. One drink led to another and then you suddenly realized you were famished. You'd been studiously avoiding chips and guacamole and deep-fried dishes for some time since you started on a healthier path, but now they were screaming your name.

You grabbed a plate, loaded it up with two chimichangas, and ladled on the rice and beans. Then you noticed the platter of gooey nachos with all your favorite toppings and heaped them on top of your already full plate.

When you woke up the next day, it felt like a Mack® truck had rolled over your body and you had the worst headache you've had in years. You ended up spending most of the day in bed and feeling terrible about your behavior. How could you have blown it so badly? You felt like you'll never get the hang of healthy eating, you'll never lose the weight, and you're hopeless. Why even try?

THE MINDSET THAT KEEPS YOU ON TRACK

To stay on track after you have a bad day when you feel like a total failure, you need to shift your mindset. This is the time to practice self-compassion, forgive yourself for your transgressions, and get right back to healthy eating. The easiest way to do this is to pretend that your best friend confessed to your behavior.

There's no way you would diss her and call her a loser. Nope. You'd cut her some slack and tell her it was totally understandable under the circumstances, and reassure her that she hadn't done any real damage. Then you'd advise her to just get back on the healthy habits bandwagon. Please treat yourself as kindly as you would treat someone you love, and move on with life.

One off-the-rails meal does not make you a worthless weak-willed individual who will never develop a healthy relationship with food. The key is to learn from the experience, practice amnesia, and get right back to your healthy life.

7. Don't Let the Meal Planning Slip

THE MINDSET THAT GETS YOU OFF TRACK

You know that one of the keys to eating healthy and staying on track is meal planning. The only way to eat healthy today is to have mapped out what you're going to eat the day before. Otherwise, you'll be living on restaurant-prepared food made with copious amounts of butter, oil, sugar, and salt. You'll also eat way too much because portion sizes are double or triple actual serving sizes.

As a result, you've gotten into the habit of devoting a few hours over the weekend to planning your meals for the week. It's a bit time consuming but it's so much easier to be healthy when you have your meals plotted ahead of time. You actually prefer bringing your lunch to work. Now you have time to take a walk since you don't have to spend time scrounging around for something to eat at lunchtime.

But last weekend turned out to be crazy busy and you just didn't have time to do your usual meal prep. The fallout has been ugly. The absence of prepared meals has led you to revert to the habits you thought you had cast off. Not so fast. This week you've eaten pepperoni pizza, huge sandwiches, and cheesy tacos for lunch, and done the drive-thru for dinner.

Now you feel like it's a lost cause. You've probably undone all your hard work from the last few months. Maybe you should just admit to yourself that you hate meal planning and you don't have time for it now that you're getting so busy. Also, you're about to go on a cruise and that's surely going to be a gorge-fest. Maybe it's time to accept that you can't do this. You'll do a juice cleanse when you get back and that will absolve you of all your sins.

THE MINDSET THAT KEEPS YOU ON TRACK

To stay on track, you need to shift your mindset. Instead of throwing in the towel, you need to be more realistic about what amount of meal prep is needed on a weekly basis. Keep in mind that the goal is to get healthy food in your body and that there are many ways to accomplish that goal.

Think about a less time-consuming way to eat healthy during busier weeks. Maybe Plan B is to buy a cooked rotisserie chicken and roast a tray of pre-cut veggies in the oven. Another option might be to go to Trader Joe's™ and buy prepared salads for lunch, and frozen entrees and vegetables for dinner. You may even opt for pre-cooked home delivered meals for the insanely busy times in life.

The point is to accommodate your food planning to your schedule and energy level. Give yourself a variety of options and just keep bobbing and weaving.

8. Experiment with a Cheat Meal

THE MINDSET THAT GETS YOU OFF TRACK

You've been sticking with a healthy diet but lately have been feeling deprived and possessed by a craving for Del Taco®. You decide that the best way to stay motivated is to give in and allow yourself a little treat. You resolve to make it a moderate splurge and only order two grilled chicken tacos.

Unfortunately, when the clerk asks you what you want, you blurt out your tried-and-true order: "# 6 Combo." This old go-to covers the waterfront of tasty food, including a beef taco, cheese quesadilla, fries, and a soda. You tell yourself that you're stemming the damage by opting for a diet soda.

You're so disgusted after that pathetic behavior that you give up on yourself and "forget" to bring lunch to the office for the rest of the week. You quickly lapse back into old fast-food habits. By Friday, you feel thoroughly defeated, and have no idea how to right the ship.

THE MINDSET THAT KEEPS YOU ON TRACK

To stay on track, you need to adjust your mindset. Tell yourself that your cheat meal was an experiment and that it's OK to try different things and fail. Consider that everyone is different. Some people can successfully enjoy a cheat meal, keep it moderate, and then pick up where they left off. For others, it's not an effective way to satisfy a craving because it leads to a sustained binge of overindulging.

Look for alternatives. You may find a recipe for a healthier version of what you love at Del Taco® and find that it is good enough to squelch the obsession. Or buy an air fryer. That might produce the crunchiness that you're looking for. Be creative and you'll discover what works for you.

9. JUDGE WEIGHT LOSS BY YOUR BODY, NOT THE SCALE

THE MINDSET THAT GETS YOU OFF TRACK

You have a love-hate relationship with the scale. You loved it when you first ditched sugar because you were losing weight fast. Seeing that number go down consistently was very motivating. You loved it less when you tried giving up all carbs. To your surprise it barely moved.

You want to lose weight desperately and don't really know any way to monitor yourself other than stepping on the dreaded scale. You know that it's not precise; things other than what you ate the day before can affect your weight. But you rely on it because it produces a number and you can't argue with it. As they say, numbers don't lie.

Last week you felt like you'd eaten like a saint, seriously curtailed restaurant dining, and been very mindful of reducing your portions. Yet when you got on the scale, the number had actually gone up almost an entire pound! You are mystified and depressed.

THE MINDSET THAT KEEPS YOU ON TRACK

To stay on track, you need to adjust your mindset. The scale is not the holy grail! In fact, it's woefully inaccurate on a day-to-day basis because there are too many variables in the mix. Hormonal changes, eating a salty meal, stress, weight training, and not having a bowel movement are just a few of the fluctuations that might impact what number the scale alights on in the morning.

The better gauge is your body. And after all, aren't changes in your body what you're really looking for? Don't you care a lot more about how you look and feel and how your clothes fit than on some random number you've picked out of the air that you decided you need to see on the scale?

Step away from the scale. Notice your energy level. Pay attention to how your clothes fit. Try on some clothes that are too small and monitor your progress that way. The important thing is that you're making progress on developing a healthy eating pattern that becomes second nature. View losing weight as just the happy byproduct of that overarching goal.

10. If You're Not Making Progress on Your Own, Get Help from a Professional

THE MINDSET THAT GETS YOU OFF TRACK

You see yourself as a person who has conquered challenging goals in life and come out on top. Your job is going well and your kids are behaving themselves by and large. You're in a pretty happy place in mid-life except for one thing.

You need to lose about 30 pounds that you've been carrying around for what seems like forever, and it's starting to bother you more every day. It's hard to ignore the fact that you now get winded climbing stairs and that your knees hurt when you walk.

One day you decide it's time to tackle the food issue and get your eating habits under control like the other areas of your life. You Google "Nutritionist" and proceed to interview three of them. They all offer different programs. The first one tells you that you will lose weight if you come in for 15-minute weigh-ins and buy her pills and protein powder. The second one recommends that you adopt a vegan diet that forsakes all animal products and saves the planet. You don't care for either of those approaches.

Your third appointment is with a Nutritionist who talks to you about gradual behavior change and focuses on reworking your eating habits. That makes a lot of sense to you and you know that's the right direction since you've tried and failed on every quick weight loss diet out there.

While you're tempted to hire her, since she sounds sensible and has reminded you of the need for outside accountability on your weight loss journey, you don't feel comfortable spending a lot of money on this, and aren't sure you have the time for the 30-minute sessions. When she follows up, you tell her that you think you can do it on your own.

You start off by purging your house of junk-food snacks and creating an elaborate meal plan for the week. That works for a few weeks and then you revert to restaurant dining and grab-n-go, and decide it's just too hard.

THE MINDSET THAT KEEPS YOU ON TRACK

To stay on track once you determine that changing your eating habits is too onerous to do solo, admit to yourself that you need help. You need a knowledgeable partner for a successful weight loss journey.

After all, you've sought psychological counseling when you needed it, even when it meant paying out of pocket. While it seems like you should be able to learn how to control what you put into your mouth without professional help, that is not the case.

You finally feel ready to acknowledge that you need the help of a professional for guidance and accountability. Even though it feels like a selfish expense, you bite the bullet and get some help.

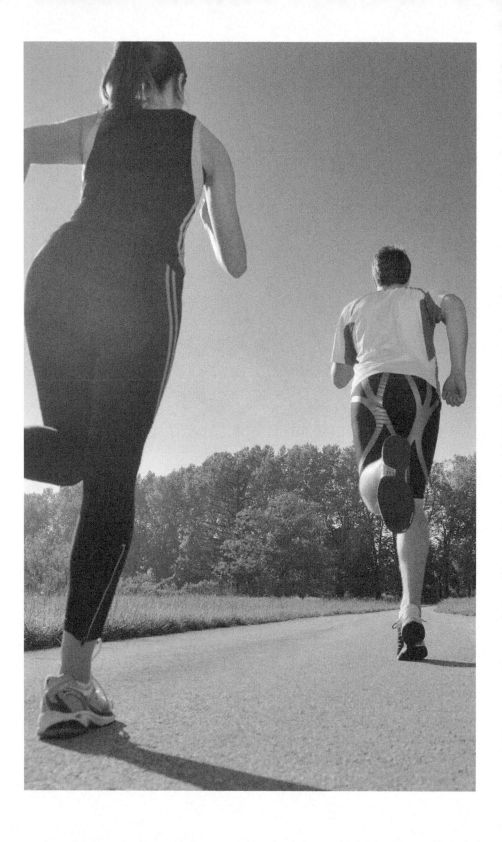

5

How to Stay on Track Forever

Does This Sound Familiar?

You're in a good place. You've finally gotten the weight off and feel so much better about yourself. You can move better and you've been able to buy a lot of cool new clothes that you love wearing.

You don't want to cycle the weight back on this time. You need to figure out what to do to stay where you are and not lose this battle yet again. This is uncharted territory. In the past, you've trusted that the weight would stay off if you just continued to pay attention to what you were eating and watched the scale. Or you rationalized that you could eat a few more treats. As it turns out, neither strategy worked.

You start brainstorming on different alternatives to stay vigilant: weigh yourself daily, continue to log your food, focus on the upcoming wedding of your nephew, ask your girlfriend to hold you accountable, try on your skinny jeans every week, keep paying for the Weight Watchers app and going to monthly meetings, etc. None of these sounds very enticing or feels very appealing.

Ultimately you decide to lighten up on yourself and just hop on the scale every Monday morning. The first two weigh-ins are fine. The third week you're up a pound but you tell yourself it's just water weight. The next week you forget to weigh yourself. Then it's Thanksgiving and you overindulge, so you're afraid to get back on the scale. You decide you need to move to a Plan B, but you're not sure what that might be.

Keeping the Weight Off

Assuming you've lost weight gradually with behavior change, congratulations! It will come as a relief to realize that you don't have to deal with that freak out moment you've had with every quick weight loss diet you've tried in the past. Those diets all required a rude readjustment back to normal life when the restrictive shackles come off and you have to make your own food decisions again. Most people are ill-equipped to cope with being thrust back into the real world after a starvation diet, and that's why they are never able to maintain a healthy weight.

This time will feel very different and that's because you've changed your relationship with food and you've acquired the skills and strategies that make it second-nature to eat healthy under normal conditions. All you have to do is keep focused on them. Clients often ask me how much they should increase their calories once they've achieved their goals. I tell them don't even think about it because you will subconsciously loosen the reins a bit anyway.

That doesn't mean you'll never go off the wagon again. Big life changes like getting married, landing a new job, moving to a different city, having a baby, or retiring, require adjustments to your eating patterns. Other likely times for the health train to derail are holidays and vacations.

Unfortunately, health is always the easiest thing to back burner because your body does not scream at you and puts up with prolonged abuse before it shows the effects of disease. When you get overwhelmed with life or there are too many demands on your time, you stop paying as much attention to eating whole foods in reasonable portions. The tug of convenience is strong and that typically means heavy reliance on restaurant prepared meals. It may take several months or even a year for you to realize that your clothes are getting uncomfortable and it isn't attributable to that mythical dryer shrinkage.

My recommendation is to periodically check in with yourself to ensure that you're still on a healthy eating track. Just make it part of your life plan. And make sure that you examine your health habits frequently enough so that you don't find you've tacked on ten new pounds of fat before it hits your radar screen that you've strayed.

Decide on Your Go-To Tools to Keep Yourself on Track

Here are my five best stay-on-track-forever tools. Read through them and make a decision about which one(s) you want to rely on to make sure that you accord healthy eating the first priority it deserves in your busy life.

TOOL #1
DON'T KEEP ANY TOO-BIG CLOTHES

Many of my clients have several sets of clothes for the different versions of themselves. I put an end to this "just in case" mentality. I don't like the idea of "go backs" in the closet because it's nothing more than a way to hedge your bets in the event that you regain the weight. That's not the mentality of someone who intends to stay healthy.

In fact, I tell my clients that as soon as any item of clothing is too big, it must leave the house. Give it to a charity or burn it on the beach, it's your choice, but don't keep it around.

What happens if you do regain a few pounds? You will immediately feel uncomfortable in your clothes and you won't have any alternative other than shopping for a bigger size; a most unpleasant experience. Not having "fat clothes" in the house will give you more incentive to stay on track.

Tool #2

Invest in an Expensive New Form-Fitting Wardrobe

This tip goes hand in hand with the prior advice. Once you've gotten to the size and shape that makes you feel proud, go out and splurge on new duds that show off the results of your hard work. You've earned the bragging rights. Buy durable classy pieces and strut your stuff.

Consider sinking your hard-earned money into quality tailored clothing as your healthier alternative to indulging in gourmet dining. Well-made clothes that hug your body also expose your sins and serve as an all-day reminder to pay attention to what you're putting in your mouth. Once you've invested in a beautiful wardrobe, you'll want to show off your threads for a long time.

Tool #3

Make Sure the Ban on Junk Food in the House Sticks

When you were laser focused on ditching the weight and super-motivated to achieve your healthy eating goals, you probably banned processed snacks from the house. But you may find that they want to weasel their way back in. First, it's just a little treat someone gave you at work and then it's just a few boxes of cookies you felt obligated to buy to support the Girl Scouts. Before you know it, your house has become a junk food haven and you realize that you've made it too easy to resume your emotional eating habits.

Sound the alarm! Call out the food police for a clean sweep before things get out of hand. Don't fool yourself. You can't portion control junk food now any better than you ever could. The ice cream knows your name and it'll use a bullhorn to get you to open the freezer and devour it just as soon as you have a weak moment.

The easiest way to successfully ostracize sweet and crunchy snacks is to avoid those aisles at the grocery store. That way, no chips or cookies jump into the cart when you're not looking. If contraband is brought in by someone else in your household, you have to be prepared to exercise your coping skills. Maybe you ask them to hide it from you. Perhaps they eat their fill and give the rest away. Or maybe you sneak it into the garbage on pick-up day and can't recall what happened to it when questioned.

Tool #4
Ensure that Meal Planning Remains Intact

One of the best weight loss tools is meal planning. In today's world we have to plan to be healthy. If you forget your lunch and you're hungry at the office, all you need do is step into the break room and plentiful free food will greet you. Drive around and you'll see a fast-food drive-thru in every shopping center. Go to a food court and you've got the world's cuisines to choose from. If you want more of a dining experience or are meeting with a client, colleague, or friend, the opportunities for restaurant dining are so abundant you'll have a hard time narrowing them down.

The point is that food is everywhere you look today. You'd have to be on a camping trip deep in the woods to escape it. And all these convenient options are very tasty because they're loaded with butter, oil, sugar, and salt. To make matters worse, they come in portion sizes suitable for an NFL linebacker who just finished his job of trying to take out the quarterback in the Super Bowl.

The bottom line is that preparing your meals in advance and taking them with you as needed, will ensure that you continue to fit into your clothes comfortably. Whereas resorting to making do with free food or restaurant prepared food will inevitably lead to not being able to zip up your jeans.

Meal planning has to remain a constant in your life. Be realistic about the amount of time you have to devote to the plan week-by-week and adjust it accordingly. Some weeks you'll have the free time and inclination to cook from scratch, and other times heating up frozen meals or throwing together a few healthy ingredients you have on hand makes more sense.

Tool #5

If Weight Creep Sets in, Go Back to Keeping a Food Diary

Research demonstrates that the most effective tool for losing weight is keeping a food diary. I prefer the MyFitnessPal© app because it allows friends, and professionals like me, to see the user's food diary. That provides both additional accountability and junk food eating deterrence.

While no one wants to keep a food diary forever, it can be very helpful to resume logging your meals when a few pounds decide to sneak back on. It will put an end to denial and reorient you if portion sizes have been creeping up. Going back to that discipline will help you quickly identify the culprit and refocus yourself on eating whole foods, while eliminating most processed foods and snacks.

Conclusion

Eating is one of the most enjoyable parts of life. This should be evident from the fact that it is the last activity we give up before we die. But most of us have been unwittingly consuming huge amounts of overly processed foods for years simply because they've become so readily available.

My purpose in writing this book is to provide a road map of the behavior change process as it applies to eating habits. This is not dieting. This is about rethinking the role food plays in your life. You've never tried this before. In the past, you've always looked for a quick fix and tried to starve off the excess pounds. But it turns out that the approach of changing your mindset is the real answer.

Now you have the skills to deal with this overabundance. You realize that a diet of whole foods is a critical component of your health and worth devoting more attention to rather than just grabbing whatever prepared food is within arm's reach or available at the drive-thru you pass on your way home.

The good news is that now that you've done the deep dive into how your brain and emotions interact with your food choices, you are officially done with dieting for the rest of your life.

Even better is that you have told food that you are the boss and have put eating in its proper place in life. Your new relationship with food is one of enjoyment in its pleasures. You're now in touch with your body's signals about hunger and fullness. You no longer eat as an emotional salve or just because there is food everywhere and you see others gobbling it down as if it's about to be rationed.

You've finally gotten the monkey off your back and are proud of the way you look. You feel so much better about yourself now that you are intentional about what you put in your mouth. It's gotten easier to choose well and resist formerly tempting snacks. You now know how to moderate portions while maintaining a normal life which allows you to continue to enjoy parties, vacations, and restaurant dining.

And if you found as you worked your way through the book, that you either weren't ready or you realized that you needed a health coach for more guidance and accountability, wait for the right time in your life and get help.

Thanks for taking the journey with me!

About the Author

Lorie Eber has had two very different careers. She spent an enjoyable 23 years as a corporate litigator for a large San Francisco law firm. Practicing law was an all-consuming profession, so at age 49 she decided she needed to switch gears in the hopes of achieving a more balanced life.

Self-discovery was the order of the day for the next 10 years as she tested the waters in various fields including Gerontology (the study of aging), working for an elder care non-profit, professional writing, and featured keynote speaking. In the course of her meanderings, she lucked into a job teaching Gerontology at Coastline College and has now created several Wellness Coaching courses that she also teaches at the school.

After a light bulb moment, Lorie realized that health and wellness coaching was well-suited to her skills and interests. But she wasn't comfortable just hanging out her shingle and offering her services. Instead, she proceeded to learn as much as she could about her chosen field so that she could be an excellent health coach.

Lorie is a Nutritionist and Weight Loss Specialist, certified in Nutrition Science by the Stanford University Center for Health Education, and is a Mayo Clinic Certified Wellness Coach. She is also credentialed by Wellcoaches School of Coaching, is an NASM Certified Personal Trainer and Nutrition Specialist, as well as a life coach.

Her one-woman business, Lorie Eber Wellness Coaching, provides one-on-one customized and personalized weight loss and healthy living coaching and support. Ms. Eber partners with her clients while they achieve healthy lifestyle changes and improve their well being. In today's food-centric culture, maintaining a healthy diet and weight is the ultimate challenge. Accountability and advice from an expert coach increase the odds of success dramatically.

Lorie is the real deal. What you see is what you get. She doesn't sugar coat things and although she can crack the whip when necessary, she also dispenses encouragement to motivate her clients, whom she gets to know on an individual basis. Everyone can change their health habits if they put in consistent effort and get the support they need for the journey.

How to Show Food Who's Boss

Even at the ripe old age of 66 Lorie walks-the-walk. That includes daily workouts of spin class or running and cardio machines, as well as strength training three times per week. She eats whole foods, lots of veggies, and pays attention to portion creep. Stress reduction is definitely a work in progress, but she (mostly) limits her work to six days a week. That may not sound like progress but given her Jewish achievement-oriented upbringing, it's still a dent in the struggle.

Lorie Eber has previously published seven books available on Amazon as paperbacks and e-Books:

1. *How to Get Out of Your Food Coma and Get Healthy*
2. *How I Escaped Legal Practice and Got Myself a Life*
3. *Why I'm Not a Fat Old Lady*
4. *How to Ditch Your Fat Clothes for Good*
5. *40 Ways to Leave Your Lover: That Would be Junk Food*
6. *How to Stay Healthy in a World Designed to Make Us Fat and Lazy*
7. *Aging Beats the Alternative and a Sense of Humor Helps*

For more information about Lorie and the lifestyle-enhancing services she offers, visit her website: www.LorieEberWellnessCoaching.com

Made in the USA
Columbia, SC
14 February 2024

31538963R00049